Rock Your Beauty Biz

Toni Thomas

ISBN: 9798704819158

DEDICATION

For Austin

CONTENTS

ACKNOWLEDGMENTS

I want to thank so many people for encouraging me to write this book and to those who helped me launch it successfully as a book and an online business course.

To Emma Lamb my marketing guru from Ninefifteen Social Media Marketing for her hard work on my marketing plan, for her amazing ideas, and her contributions to the marketing section of this book and the online course. To Kerry Metcalfe from KMedia for her truly amazing email marketing approach that helped to get this book and the online course the exposure it deserved. To my entire marketing team, I am blessed to have you in my life assisting me on this journey to help beauty industry professionals achieve their full potential.

To my family and friends who encouraged me to keep working even in the face of the darkest days of my life, without your support I would not be able to continue to do what I am passionate about.

To my husband Rob Thomas for always supporting my endeavors and for having the faith in me that I would get one more book to the publisher.

YOUR BEAUTY BIZ

Are you ready to **Rock Your Beauty Business**?

Are you ready to launch a breakout business this year that takes your professional business to a new level of success?

The global beauty industry is projected to reach more than $750 billion by 2026 and as a beauty industry professional, you are perfectly placed to be a part of this growing industry.

Your business is ready to **skyrocket**!

Are you ready for the **launch**?

This book was designed for all beauty industry professionals and is structured for the following professions: hairstylists, colorists, barbers, estheticians, aestheticians, makeup artists, massage therapists, reflexologists, nail technicians, aromatherapists, beauty product sales, fashion photographers, wardrobe stylists and all beauty industry professionals.

In this book, I want to share how I built a thriving international beauty business.

"I'm sharing what I learned from my experience in my own beauty business. I know how difficult it can be to build a successful beauty business and the struggles that come from launching your new career. It wasn't easy for me; it was a long journey of discovery that took me years to figure out how to apply just the right techniques to build my successful beauty career."

But I did it and so can **you**...

I took my **BIG** dreams and started **small**; I applied a series of easy strategies that allowed me to build a thriving career in the beauty industry...

My **small** and consistent approach to my business launched a **BIG** career. I now teach beauty courses all over the world, I run a successful online beauty academy, I am the author of seven beauty industry books, I am the creative director for a fashion and beauty magazine, and best of all I attend New York Fashion Week every year as an invited makeup artist and guest beauty blogger! I also run a successful on-location makeup team and work in my salon a few days per month as an esthetician.

I'm busy but I **love** what I do, and it means I work when I want, where I want, with who I want, and I get to travel the world.

My **BIG** dreams started with **small** techniques that anyone can duplicate, and I want to share them with you so you can achieve your dreams and live the life you have always wanted.

Wouldn't you like to have a career that takes you beyond your wildest dreams and gives you a life filled with **passion, purpose,** and **intention**?

This beauty business blueprint can be applied to any professional beauty business and if done properly can give you the **successful** beauty business you have always wanted.

Don't you think it's time to start **rocking** your beauty business?

It took me years and years to perfect my strategies, but it will take you a short time to learn my techniques. Within a few weeks of completing this book, you will have the knowledge to implement what you've learned and take your career to a new level of success.

This will be your **cheat sheet** to success.

In this groundbreaking **book** you'll learn:

* How to build a business plan in 5 days.

* How to launch an online portfolio with no money.

* How to gain a strong presence and get instant credibility in your industry.

* How to build relationships that matter and get you lasting results.

* How to get new clients, and how to make a bigger profit from your existing clientele.

* How to sell your beauty products without feeling pushy or salesy.

* How to create your own marketing blueprint designed exclusively for you.

* How to get amazing results on a small budget.

* How to become a consistent marketer with a plan that works.

* How to charge higher prices for your services and have your customers thank you and refer their friends and family.

I am excited to take you on a journey of discovery where you will learn how to launch or relaunch your professional beauty business and live the life you have always wanted.

Start **small** think **BIG**.

You deserve it...

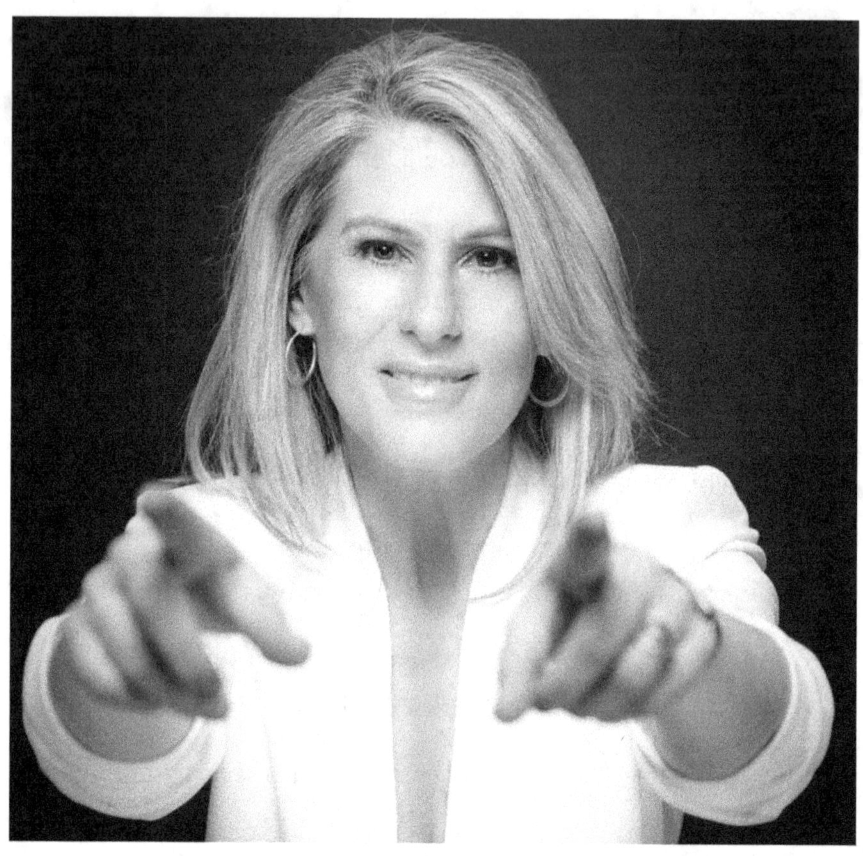

YOUR JOURNEY

Becoming a successful beauty industry professional takes a well thought out plan, career decisions filled with intention, and the drive to take action in your business. This book was created for every beauty professional who is looking to achieve a successful career and is ready to gain the knowledge, utilize the tools, and take advantage of the provided resources to help you reach the top of your industry.

And isn't the top where all of us would like to be?

This is a comprehensive **blueprint** to assist you while you build your new business or re-launch your career. This is a complete guide to help you find your niche market and get a good understanding of ways to market in a fashion that allows your creative side to flow through. From the onset of your business, you will need a plan so powerful that no one can dissuade you from your dream career, not even you.

Yes, you heard that right, not even you!

By nature, we tend to be our biggest critic and we have the potential to quit doing that which is hard right before we give it time to become a success. Some of this is from lack of patience and some from fear of success. As with any new business, the building period takes time and requires a great deal of perseverance.

This book will help you to strategize your business and hopefully inspire the positive actions you need to take to launch your career and your beauty business. It will also provide many resources to assist you in the age of fast-changing technology, social media marketing, and the global economy. This book is a working tool and for your success you must be involved and begin implementing the techniques you learn.

I'm not here to waste your time I'm here to help you implement strategies that you can start doing today and reap the rewards tomorrow. These strategies work if you are willing to work! I want you to take this **blueprint** and launch your marketing as soon as possible. Your success will depend on your decision to apply the techniques and strategies that I have mapped out for you.

Note to the reader

"Becoming a beauty professional is the easy part of your journey, creating your new business is going to be the hard part. I encourage you to take your time, learn the techniques, implement the strategies, and follow the business-building formulas I have created to execute your beauty business with purpose and intention. You are heading into your new adventure as an entrepreneur and the future looks bright and beautiful."

-Toni Thomas

Beauty Business Guru and Founder of The Beauty Academy

YOUR PLAN

Do you have a business plan?

Did you know you can create one in 5 days or less?

Knowing what your options are in your industry is the very first step in your success and understanding how to implement your plan is the key to what will separate you from the average. In this life, we are what we choose to become, and your career options are wide open as a beauty professional.

Want to know the secret is to become a great beauty professional?

Confidence is the key to your future success followed by a well thought out plan that you implement and follow. Once you begin to feel confident in your profession you will need to take your skills and showcase the results to the world around you. You are the only one who can find and market to your future clients and lead them to your services and products. Confidence is the path to your business success.

Do you know the who, what, when, and where?

To get a closer look at your business plan options you will first need to understand the who, the what, the when, and where of your business. To do this you will need to describe who you are as a beauty professional, such as your skill level and the market you are trying to target. What your new business does, such as techniques and special skills you possess. You will need to know when you will be open for business, what the hours of operation are and where your business is going to be located. This could include mobile services as well as a studio service. Is your new business going to be a local or global business and if it's global how far are you willing to travel? In addition, you will need to determine what your short and long-term goals are for your business future. Where do you see your business headed in 1 to 3 years and in 5 to 10 years?

As a beauty professional it is your job to help clients on many occasions, you are after all in the beauty business. Even as a barber you are not only cutting hair, but you are helping someone to feel good about their appearance. As a photographer you give your clients memories, as a makeup artist, you make sure their future memories look beautiful for future generations to enjoy. Through your skills, you give others confidence. You are a **wizard** who empowers others by giving them confidence in who they are. Have you ever seen a person who has emerged from a salon or spa or a photoshoot who didn't walk with a little more pep in their step? You made them feel good! This is your special skill; you make others feel good! Many beauty industry professionals help others by doing makeovers with their clients who want to update their everyday look. You might even specialize in niche markets that assist people in learning how to correct or hide defects. You are the problem solver, and everyone has problems they want solved.

Be a Wizard with a Plan

You are a **wizard**, and with the magic skills that you possess, you help people. The most successful professionals are those who help others solve problems and as a beauty professional you have all the skills to do just that.

It is also your job to have a solid business plan in place before you launch your business. Whatever you decide to do with your career you are the only one who can choose the market you want to target. You and only you can determine your skill level and what you are capable of. You are the person who is going to create your business plan and set into motion the strategies to make your plan a complete success. Once you begin to implement your plan the tough part will be to stick to your plan and execute it with dedicated precision.

The Plan

Your 5-day business plan challenge when complete will be a working document and can be updated as you determine what is working for your business and what might not be working. One thing's for sure, building your plan is the first step to a solid footing in your new career. The vision for your business has to be crystal clear for you to pursue your dream of becoming a successful beauty industry professional.

Let's Build Your Plan in 5 Days

Are you ready to start creating your business plan?

Are you ready to join the 5-Day Beauty Biz Plan challenge?

I am going to walk you through the 5-day business plan challenge and help you as you create your simple but effective plan to launch your beauty biz with ease and confidence.

Day 1

1. Download a Business Plan Template

2. Join the Rock Your Beauty Biz Facebook group online

In the Rock Your Beauty Business Facebook group, we will be doing live working sessions together where I will host our challenge, and where you will be submitting your work on a few of the challenges. This group is also a great place to ask questions, find answers, and discuss roadblocks you have in your current business or future business with fellow beauty professionals who have been there before you.

3. Write Your Business Summary

Get a notebook. You are going to need a 3-divider notebook or something similar to write in and a pen or pencil to start mapping your business plan. This is a requirement. You will use this notebook for future chapters in this beauty business course. The first step to a good business plan is to write your business summary.

A business **summary** should be included in the beauty business plan to explain the entire idea and concept. It should summarize the entire business plan in a short, concise but all-encompassing format. Assume your most important readers will read only this section that is why it should be 5-10% of the size of the entire business plan and written in the same sequence as the business plan. It usually contains a brief statement of the proposal covered, background information, and the main conclusion. Write your story or your dream on paper.

4. Write Your Business Structure

Describe your business in great detail, the goal is to get it all out on paper so you have a **blueprint** of your ideas and where you can begin to weed out things that may not fit into your biz structure.

A beauty business plan must include information regarding the kind of business entity you want for your start-up. The beauty industry accommodates small businesses as well as big chains. Therefore, before starting the beauty business plan, it is important for you to decide on a model, scale, and ownership structure for the business.

Is your business, sole proprietorship or a partnership? Include your company name or proposed name, the address and contact information, as well as your **business structure** (sole proprietorship, LLC, LLP, etc.). State the purpose of your organization and describe your **customer service philosophy** this is essential. Think about how you want to operate your business. If your business is a mobile salon or spa or an on-location beauty business, then make sure you add a PO Box address or your home address.

Start Dreaming!

Day 2

Step 1: What Services Will You Offer?

There are many different kinds of services that you can offer. The broad categories are hair care, nail care, skincare, makeup, barbering, lashes, waxing, spray tans, reflexology, massage therapy, etc... You must choose any one or more of the categories according to your expertise and the trends that are popular in your area. However, you have to provide the most basic services as the maximum number of customers seek them. Once you have decided on all the services, write them down in detail. Also, elaborate on what benefits your clients will get and how much each service will cost. Some of the services you can offer are:

- **Hair:** Haircut, relaxers, perms, color, shampoo, conditioning, curling, reconstructing, eyebrows, treatment, hair spa, hair removal.
- **Nails:** Manicure, pedicure, polish, nail sculpture, Acrylic nail application, nail art, etc.
- **Skincare:** Facial, waxing, massage, tan removing, spa, hydrotherapy body piercing, exfoliation.
- **Makeup:** Bridal makeup, party makeover, makeovers, prom makeup.
- **Lashes:** Extensions, tinting, lifting.

You need to decide what's on the menu, literally. What **services** do you intend to offer to your clientele? And how are they different than the ones offered by your competition?

Here's where you will **map** out the services you will provide, and whether you will include other add on services.

This section of your business plan should also include customer service aspects such as:

- How the customer experience will differ from your competitors' services.
- How you plan to maximize customer experiences.
- Whether you will cater to the upscale end of the market by taking reservations for personalized services or serve walk-ins.

Step 2: Your Market

Describe your target market including your market demographics (age, income) and market growth. Research the age group you're targeting as well as what are the current trends being followed by that age group. Include tables and charts that show your market growth. A beauty business should include all genders and age groups. Your target audience can be:

- Working Professionals
- Working Men
- Working Women
- College Students
- Stay-at-home-moms
- Teens
- Brides
- Children

Each group will require a different type of service. List each individual section of your target market and what services they would require as part of the market study.

Your target market is a description of who's going to buy your services. In this section, try to be as specific as possible. If you define your target market too broadly in the hopes of appealing to more potential clients, you can run the risk of diluting the uniqueness of your services and branding that sets you apart from your competitors.

Here are some questions you can ask yourself that will help you home in on your target market:

1. Are your target clients male, female, or both?
2. Will you offer high-end services? What's the range of your services?
3. How old are your target clients?
4. Where do they live?
5. Is geography a factor?
6. Is ethnicity a factor?
7. What do your target clients do for a living?
8. How much money do they make? (This can be an important factor that weighs into your assessment of what the clientele in your area can afford and will determine the prices you set for your services.)
9. What other aspects of their lives matter? Are they moms, dads, singles, teens, or grandparents?
10. Is the community where you're working affluent? Middle class? Blue-collar?

Day 3

Step 1: Your Strategy

Focus on certain services and make an estimate of your sales and cost for those services. Define the milestones in your business with specific dates or time periods. Decide what your strategy for the implementation is going to be and how you're going to spread the word once you start your business. Brand promotion is very important in the beauty salon business. The success of any budding beauty business depends on a core group of clients. Plan ahead for your marketing strategy. You must decide and create the content you will be using for marketing beforehand and the advertising and business strategies must be part of the beauty business plan.

Step 2: Your Staff

Proper planning with respect to manpower is one of the most challenging issues in starting a beauty business. Will you have a staff or will it, just be you? Will it be you but with a front desk staff person? Either way, employees are the front-line representatives of your business. Their talent and skill, as well as their people skills, will influence every aspect of the business. The main responsibilities in any beauty business depend on the kind of services the staff will provide. Some of the common ones are:

- Salon manager
- Hairstylist
- Cosmetologist
- Receptionist
- Manicurist
- Salon assistants

Name and describe in detail the main members of your team and what their responsibilities will be. List the gaps in management if there are any and show how they will be addressed. This will give you a better idea of the personnel required before you start and what each member is required to do.

Even if you are flying solo in your new business one of the hardest hurdles is to work all the aspects of the business without any help. You are good at your craft and you know how to provide quality services, sell products, and give great customer service and experiences. But do you know how to do all the rest of the back office skills required for a truly successful business? If not, then it's time to consider farming out certain aspects of your business for ultimate success.

These back-office duties can literally be given to other individuals who have the time and experience to help you run a successful beauty business.

- **Virtual receptionist:** (booking appointments, fielding emails, answering calls, running the website, managing the booking app)
- **Social media marketer**: (managing social media sites, managing monthly marketing emails, etc...)
- **Virtual bookkeeper:** (payroll, accounting, etc...)
- **Personal assistant:** (running errands, buying inventory, managing the business)
- **Cleaner:** (salon cleaning, laundry, etc...)

Day 4

Step 1: The Finances

No one wants to talk about money but without it, you can't start a business that will succeed.

The first thing you will need to figure out before starting a business is where will the start-up and operational money come from? Do you have it in savings, will you have investors, will you take out a loan? Knowing where you stand financially is the only way to guarantee your long-term success.

According to the SBA, about half of all new establishments survive five years or more, and about a third survive 10 years or more. In many instances, a business's failure to survive is due to poor planning and lack of funds to sustain it through its first few years of operation.

That's why it's imperative to figure out how much money you need to get started, where it will be coming from, what you will be spending it on, and how long it will take you to earn it back. What will your return on investment be or what is your ROI?

Finance is the most important part of any business. You should aim to be as specific as you can when it comes to your finances, which will include describing your financial strategy and how it will support your projected growth. Evaluating the overall costs involved in the services should give you effective pricing for the services you're going to provide. Include a break-even analysis that shows risks as a matter of fixed and variable costs and include a detailed projected profit or loss and balance sheets.

Estimate your liquid fund requirements to start your business. Before you actually start running the salon, you must purchase all the products, materials, and equipment required for the services you're providing.

Write down what the services are and what the raw materials and equipment are required for them.

For example:

- Haircutting: Oil, gel, shampoo, scissors, combs, brushes.
- Highlights: Hair dye, foil, brush, gloves, shampoo, conditioner.
- Hairstyling: Oil, gel, hairbrushes, and combs, blow dryers, curler, straightener.

You must also decide where the funding for your business will come from, whether in the form of bank loans, self-funding, and small business grants. You can finance your business by putting in the funds yourself or by borrowing money from family or friends willing to invest in your business. Whether you're borrowing money through a traditional bank loan or have teamed up with investors, you need to figure out how much money you need to get started. Research the paths for each and come to a decision about which one is suitable for you. There can however be situations when funding is difficult to seek and that is when you need to learn the essentials of how to open a salon with no money or with limited funds to get started and witness the business grow slowly but steadily.

Create a financial summary section in your business plan that includes projected financial statements spanning at least three years, or until you estimate the business will be cash-flow positive. Include all expected startup expenses based on your experience and list potential sources of initial funding. Estimate how many clients you will serve and how quickly your client base will grow, then base your revenue and direct cost estimates on these numbers.

Here are some other things to consider:

- Calculate your monthly expenses, including rent, licensing, training, payroll, supplies, and an emergency fund.
- Calculate how much of a cushion you have in savings and how much you absolutely must make each month to stay in business.
- Figure out how much you'll charge for services. To do this, estimate how many services you might perform in a week and figure out how much you'll need to charge in order for you to make a net profit. Try using a price point that is both fair for your clients and prosperous for you. Also, find out what other salons in your area charge so you can keep your prices competitive.
- Consult a certified public accountant (CPA) to help you estimate your taxes.

You might want to check out a business start-up cost calculator for a list of other items you may want to include in your financial summary.

Day 5

Step 1: Create a Marketing Plan, a Social Media Marketing Plan, and an Initial Marketing Budget

Describing how you intend to effectively market your beauty business is a crucial part of your business plan. In fact, the **marketing blueprint** you develop now can help you achieve your business goals.

Outline all the methods and outlets you plan to use to promote your beauty business: email marketing, your website; social networks like Facebook, Twitter, Pinterest, and Instagram; and directory sites like Yelp and Google, and other outlets. Research whether local newspapers, radio stations, or community magazines would effectively promote your services. Assess whether or not you want to offer membership and or loyalty programs.

We will go into your marketing plan further on in this workshop but know that without an effective marketing strategy you will struggle in your business.

Step 2: Understand the Commitment

Your commitment to your marketing plan might be the single most important aspect of your business. You may have the talent and you may have a following but without consistently marketing your business and your brand you will never have the business you dream of.

The Bottom Line

The bottom line here is that, if you can offer unique services, provide superior customer service, and build strong personal relationships your prospective clients will want to do business with you and current clients will refer you to their friends. Your business plan is only as good as your ability to build and maintain relationships.

YOUR PORTFOLIO

Did you know you can launch an online portfolio with no money?

You absolutely can and it will give your business instant credibility.

How important is it to build your portfolio?

As far as your business goes it is one of the most important elements for your success as a beauty professional. Building your portfolio is not only critical, but it is also expected in today's world of photo-driven social media marketing. Clients no longer accept that you are the best; they want to see that you are the best and they want to know that you have taken the time to create a look-book for them to review. A place where they can see your work and the results of your profession.

Your portfolio must contain your top work and have the ability to showcase your talents in a number of ways. If you are a well-rounded beauty professional, you may need to have more than one look-book. If you are working as a niche artist your potential clients will want to check out your signature looks. You may have prom girls and their mothers that just want to see your trendy prom looks. You might also need a look-book for the everyday woman looking for a makeover session and lessons. Don't forget about your specialty looks, these will need to be showcased as well. You can see where this is going, it means that if I am your customer, I don't want to slog through hundreds of pictures looking for the one photo of what I want. I expect you the professional to have it created and have it separated into categories so I can easily access and find the look I want. If you are in esthetics or reflexology it isn't as easy to showcase photos of your work, but you still need to resonate with your audience. Use before and after photos or more importantly use video to show your modalities in action.

How to create your online portfolio instantly

In today's market, you no longer carry around a physical portfolio with your pictures inside, instead, you are pulling out your smartphone or tablet to share your online portfolio. You may also be sending your potential clients a link to your portfolio website or a web link before you ever meet them in person. In today's technology-based world it will be expected that you have an online portfolio filled with your work that is relevant to the look they are trying to achieve.

Building your online portfolio can be done in less than 5 minutes. Your portfolio will require more than just your image gallery; it will also be the place where you house your online resume and your online biography with a current photograph of you. Even if you are just starting out in your beauty business you will need to create your biography. Your bio should contain some key facts about yourself such as your education and your certified skill level or whether you are a self-taught well-seasoned professional. It should also contain a brief background on you and your interests. Make it fun and exciting with just a touch of personal info. Talking about your family is acceptable to a point but it should really just be the professional details about you and your profession along with any competitions you have entered, any fashion shows you worked, any awards you have received, and any volunteer work that directly relates to your career.

Instagram Portfolio

One of the best portfolio sites is creating an Instagram Business Page and doing all the right things to make it not only a place where you create your portfolio but if done properly you can use it as your greatest marketing tool. You need to start with a well written Instagram profile bio, create high-quality photos, and use hashtags that work and can give you an Instagram portfolio that attracts clients and becomes one of your best business tools.

We will cover more about your Instagram page in the marketing section of this course.

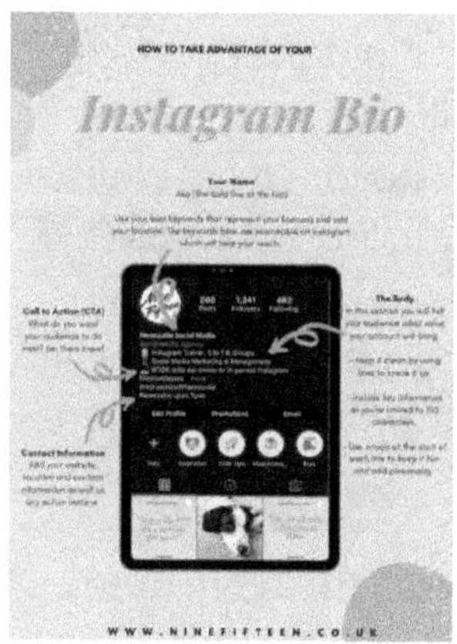

Before & After Photos

You are in charge of capturing your portfolio images and in so doing you will need to make sure to photograph each and every one of your practice models as well as you're paying customers. This will require a good quality camera or a smartphone that lets you generate quality pictures. I recommend taking a short class on photography to learn how to use your camera or your phone to capture the best photos possible. If you are on a budget, then utilize YouTube to watch free videos on capturing and editing your photos for your online look-book. I also recommend using a good online photo editor to edit and size your pictures to give them a polished look.

No surprise, lighting is the #1 issue with a lot of photos. You've spent a lot of time on your work, and you want it to look its best in your photographs. Invest in a ring light that can give you good lighting for every shot you take.

Avoid harsh light. Don't shine a light bulb onto the subject's face: you'll get a glare in the photo and the intensity of the light will diffuse the color you've worked so hard on.

Natural light is by far your best choice but avoid direct sunlight as it can have a similar effect as a bright light bulb. Instead, try morning or evening light, a cloudy day (if you're outside), or simply an indoor shot in a room with a large window that lets in a fair amount of indirect sunlight.

If you're taking a shot indoors, you can also use an umbrella or piece of white cardboard to diffuse light from a fluorescent or incandescent light bulb. Ring lights are great but can be harsh. Use a plain backdrop to get the best photos and always ask your client if you can share their image. Never take it for granted that they have agreed to their image being shared.

Note: A flash on a camera is the equivalent of shining an extremely bright light right in your face as the picture is captured. Try to avoid using a flash when photographing your work.

Before and after photos are your best marketing tool...

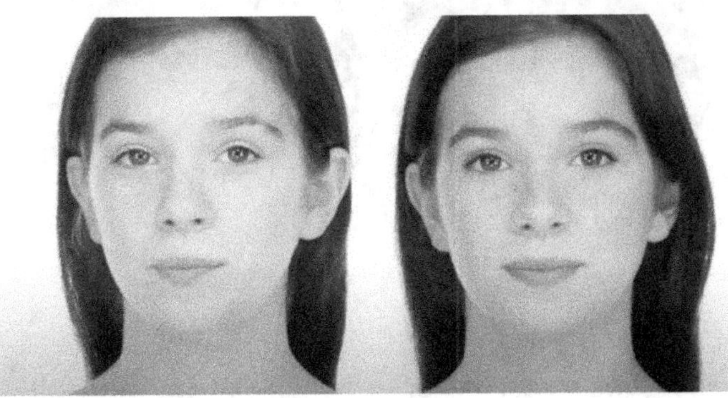

Professional Photography

Don't forget if you are working in an environment where a professional photographer will be taking photos to make sure to exchange business cards and ask that any photos of the clients be shared with you for your business portfolio. He or she may be happy to share their photos as long as you credit their work with each photo you use and send business their way. This is a win-win scenario for both you and the photographer. You get high-quality pictures, and they get exposure in your online presence. You might also try to bring in a professional photographer for important events you are working on, offer to trade services in exchange for their high-quality photos. You might have to pay for their time to be there, but you might be able to get some incredible images to use in your portfolio. It is never beneath you to try and negotiate with your fellow professionals. We are all in the business of marketing ourselves. Give something of value in exchange for something of value. Use images of yourself working on clients. These are so powerful. They tell the story of you and your business from an insider's look.

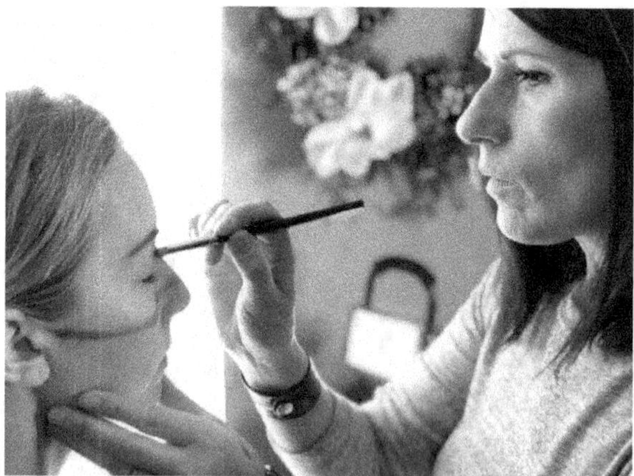

Release Forms

You are also in charge of making sure that each person you photograph will allow you to use his or her image in your portfolio.

I recommend that you carry release forms for everyone you ask to photograph. This way if your client agrees to let you use their image it can be used for your online business page and will not cause any legal problems for you in the future.

It is your responsibility to treat your business as a legal entity and to take all the precautions that any professional would.

Time is Money

You are now a professional beauty industry professional and your time is valuable. It will be up to you to always charge rates that are comparable to your skills. Do not let others devalue your work by negotiating you into a rate that doesn't make business sense. You are a freelance makeup artist, and your skills are needed and wanted by many. Stick to your listed prices and do not negotiate terms that leave you feeling short. Your self-confidence will guide you in the process of charging the rates you know are worth your time. Always check in with fellow makeup artists to gauge price comparable.

Portfolio Sites

Instagram is a great place to keep a record of your portfolio and easy for many people to find images of your work. But note that using Instagram as your portfolio site means you must only upload images of your work and leave personal posts out.

Other Portfolio Sites

www.bigblackbag.com

www.foliosnap.com

www.viewbook.com

YOUR SUCCESS

Your character

Character determines that which generates your success. We build our character over time and through the lessons we learn in life. Not everyone chooses to go in a positive direction and not everyone understands the value of having a good character. But make no mistake your character or lack of will play an important role in building and maintaining your business.

What does have a good character have to do with your professional beauty business?

It's **everything**

A strong character has everything to do with your business and your future success. Good character is a reflection of many good personal traits and you as a beauty professional need to encompass a vast majority of these traits.

Character Definition

The dictionary defines character as *"the mental and moral qualities distinctive to an individual."*

Abraham Lincoln said, "Reputation is the shadow. Character is the tree." Having a strong character is doing the right thing because it is the right thing to do.

Good character means a solid foundation and an understanding of who you are and what your value system is. It encompasses a strong work ethic followed by living your life in a standard that reflects positively on you and others. It is the foundation of choosing to be inherently good by nature even when it's easier to do otherwise. It is in fact a reflection of the choices we make in the hard parts of our lives that bring about positive results in our future. Each of us has the ability to live our life with a good and strong character, and the result of your decision to live your life with good character will be lasting relationships that are built on trust.

Discretion

As a working beauty professional in the beauty industry, working closely with others is a huge part of your job. This means often times you will hear things that others say to co-workers and other people in a studio setting. You will be told things you may not really want to know, and you will be trusted with the knowledge given freely to you by clients and customers. I have found in this industry that when working closely with clients they tend to trust in you with some of their intimate life details. It's not your place to repeat their stories nor for you to judge their personality based on the things they tell you. When working so closely with others while in close proximity it is a distinction of your character to hold true to your value set and stay focused on the job at hand. You are the first and last stop in the transfer of information.

As a working beauty professional, you may come into contact with a wide variety of personalities and at times not every one of those individuals will be looking out for you and your best interest. It is up to you to protect your good character by only taking jobs that feel right to you. That being said I am trying to tell you that your career should be earned through mutual trust and respect. Do unto others, as you would have them do unto you. Act professionally at all times and keep discretion close to your business model.

This will bring you a great deal of respect in your career not only by your peers but by your clients as well.

Your Credibility

Building your credibility in the beauty industry is important and it isn't that hard to get if you follow a few rules that will set you apart from your competitors. You get it instantly if you market your services and begin helping others solve their problems. As I said before, "solving problems is your #1 goal."

How do you build your credibility?

I have three rules I personally follow as a beauty industry professional and if you are offering services or products to clients or customers you need to believe that these three rules apply to your business framework as well.

If you are offering products or services in your beauty industry career you need to hear this!

1. We all want solutions to our problems.

2. We all want an enjoyable customer experience.

3. We all want to know you have a purpose or a mission we can believe in.

The truth is consumers don't come to you for your products or services they come to you for **YOU**! We are human and being human means, we love to feel connected. You are the reason your business is successful. It is not the people around you who make you successful or the products and services you offer. They come to you for you!

How do I apply these rules?

When I decided to build up my credibility in my industry, I wrote a book that helped women learn some beauty secrets. I showed them how to do some easy makeup techniques that they could apply to their everyday makeup routine and achieve a flawless-looking makeup that lasted all day. They had a problem and I helped to solve it.

I use the 3-rule framework in my business every day and you should too.

1. Show others how to solve their problems.

2. Give excellent customer service and always be discrete.

3. Share your purpose. Let your customers be a part of your purpose, they are thrilled to help others just as you are helping them.

You Can Solve Problems

You can solve problems; they don't even need to be problems that are in your industry.

You can do short videos that show others how to get salon results at home. You can do live workshops on an at-home process. You can deliver at-home products in person. You can do short photo or video tutorials. You can post before and after photos!

You are the only one who can build your credibility, videos and photos are a great way to become an industry leader in your community. Create a Facebook group, invite your potential clients, friends, and relatives to the group, and start sharing tips and tricks. Even a 3-minute video can help build your credibility if you are helping others solve a problem. You don't even need to solve a problem in your area of expertise.

Get creative! I suggest starting **simple**. Try teaching your new group how to wrap a scarf in 4 different ways or teach 6 ways to style black jeans or how to make an easy holiday Christmas ornament with their kids! All of these things begin giving you instant credibility and will start to gain you a following, and in the process, you are helping others solve problems. We are all looking for inspiration in our lives and you can give it to them. This is how you get instant credibility.

Consistent content, solving problems, and inspiring others while you share your mission or your passion!

How do you maintain long term credibility?

Show up on time and be a professional! **Always! Always! Always!**

I can't stress enough how important it is to show up on time, be a professional, and follow up with every client and customer...

Marketing and building your professional presence may be the most time-consuming part of your new business but in this industry having a strong presence will give you the edge over your competitors.

What does building your professional presence really mean?

In essence, you are building your brand and creating your image. It means that you are opening the doors of your business and you have hung out your open sign.

One of the first things you will need to determine is whether you are going to be a local beauty professional or a global beauty professional. More often than not one leads to the other. You may start small in your local community building your business, honing your skills, and networking with community members. If you are motivated and ambitious you may find yourself accepting opportunities farther away from your local market, maybe accepting jobs for professional photoshoots. If you are successful and ambitious you may find yourself becoming a jet-set entrepreneur, and make no mistake about it, when you decide to become a professional beauty business entrepreneur you have the potential to work just about anywhere.

Your Social Media Marketing Plan

Get your social networking skills on because now is the time to start thinking about your marketing plan. This is a critical time in your career to make people aware of your business. Using social media is a great way to get started on your marketing plan and building your professional presence.

One of the first things you need to do is **clean up** all of your current social media sites. You may think that your personal and professional image will never cross over or that what you have posted on your sites in the past will have no effect on the future of your business. Think again, you have just opened up your doors for more scrutiny than you ever imagined and if you think your potential clients are not out doing their homework on you then you would be very wrong. You are now a professional and that means your personal image and professional image are merged into one. Time to clean up your accounts and start acting like the professional you are.

Your professional presence will be determined by your ability to give practical value to your potential customers. You will only be able to market that which provides benefit and value to others. You are about to enter the world of marketing.

Every opportunity is a stepping-stone so remember at all times to look your very best. You are the product of what you are trying to sell, and the brand of your work is on your face and in the clothes, you choose to wear. Your personal image is very important when presenting yourself to your clients. People will associate your wardrobe with your skills, this may not be fair, but it is how the world works, so be prepared to create a personal style to go along with your beauty business. Always be professional and look the part. If you struggle with how to dress for your new business, try consulting YouTube channels that focus on stylists who dress and style beauty professionals and people who are working in the beauty industry.

Your Collaborations

Are you collaborating with other beauty industry professionals? I personally do this all the time. It costs me little money and a small amount of my time, but the results are huge! Did you hear me the results are **HUGE...?**

Collaborations give you outcomes that you can't buy.

If you are a stylist try working with makeup artists and photographers on stylized photo shoots. This gets you not only exposure through your social sites, but it gets you exposure on their social sites. The results of creative collaborations can be one of your best business decisions.

I personally have worked on several creative collaborations and these collaborations have garnered me a great deal of success in my makeup artistry career. Once you start working with other talented creatives and you show up as a professional, on time, and ready to work you will start to get referrals for paid work as well as get invitations to large-scale projects.

Because of my willingness to do non-paid **collaborations** with other talented photographers, stylists, models, and artists I am now invited to NYFW every season. I am invited to work on editorial magazine photoshoots, and I have been hired by NBC News and FOX news to work on-location gigs. Collaborating is all a part of building relationships and relationships mean everything in the beauty industry.

"I would rather work with a few people who are committed than a hundred people who are interested. The results of committed far outweigh the results of interested."

- Toni Thomas

YOUR WORTH

What is your worth in this industry?

As a beauty industry professional one of the most difficult tasks is to determine your value and worth. It is difficult but can easily be accomplished by doing your research and due diligence. You can start your research by going online to a site called o*net online at onetonline.org to see what others are earning in this field all across the US.

O*net says that the median wage for beauty professionals in the US is about $21.30 per hour or $44,310 per year. This is a beginning income in the beauty industry, and it can be achieved easily if you apply yourself to your profession. However, it is not a true reflection of what can be made if you are driven and committed to your profession and are willing to learn the strategies and implement a plan that has purpose and outcomes. I know many beauty industry leaders who make 6 figures or more and some who make **WAY** more!

But how do you really determine how much to charge per hour, per service, or by the client?

You and only you can determine your **monetary** value. You build up your **worth** as you build up your skills and your professional presence. This is how we determine our value. **Time is money** as we have already discussed so you want to be very careful not to devalue your services by not charging appropriately for your time. You can easily do this by doing your homework and research.

Grab your notebook and or planner and start asking a few questions.

- What are your competitors charging?
- How good are their services and what is their reputation in the industry?
- Do they service walk-in clients, or do they know how to maintain clients and get referrals?
- What scale are they using to determine their worth and how can you scale your business?
- What are your competitors doing to promote their business?
- Do they give value and are they solving problems while also providing great customer service?

Answer these questions and then set your base prices with add on prices to give your customers and clients options. But as I said before you should be keeping your service menu simple and easy to read.

There are stages to building your value and determining your monetary worth. Try to look at the big picture, not the short-term quick fix. If this is your business and your long-term career goals are to become a full-time beauty professional, then building your business professionally will begin with you working in your field of expertise as much and as often as possible. You should be working and practicing your craft each and every day. If you are not doing hands-on applications every day, then you need to stay in the know by researching and reading or taking continuing education courses. Follow all the professionals who you admire that are making it happen in their beauty industry careers. Follow those professionals who have the same value system as you and are working toward the same goals. Stay connected to the fashion and beauty industry and follow all the current trends. Determine what trends are long lasting and what trends are about to be up and coming. It is up to you to create the professional world you want to be a part of and to determine your value and worth for your time and services. Time is money!

Stage One

The first stage is getting your feet wet, or more likely getting familiar with how this industry really works. It is a time of building your network, practicing your skills, and gaining confidence in your abilities. This is where you practice your craft every day and start building your **business acumen**. You will begin to get a feel for your professional surroundings to learn how to assert your monetary value. You are building your plan, your presence, and your knowledge to gain a reputable and solid presence in the beauty industry. This stage is your 1-3 year phase and will require you to be well prepared for every person who will try and get more for less. It is also the period in your career that will require you to have a strong and sensible backbone, to overcome your doubts about what to charge for your services. It is when you will do your research and determine your worth. It is the period of your business when you practice your skills each and every day and seek out knowledge in your industry. It is the opportune time for you to volunteer your time and services, attend as many professional meetings as possible, and create a buzz about your new business. You will be the person who will share your enthusiasm with others and get the media talking about you. You are the professional so be on your game and be the best.

Stage Two

You are the only one who can create value in your business, and it is worth your time to create a **monetary value** that is above reproach. A true professional knows that their time and expertise is valuable. If you are traveling to clients your time is even more valuable and the costs associated with this need to be reimbursed. You need to have an income that substantiates your true professionalism and if anyone tells you they can get the same services elsewhere for a better price it is your responsibility to remind them that your services are worth the prices you are advertising.

Why?

Because they are getting you and you know your value and you need to translate to them how valuable you are.

How?

Direct them to all your social sites, show them your portfolio, get them the link to your website, and always be a professional in every aspect of your life.

Do not devalue yourself to fit into the mass mold.

It is up to you to create your value for the profession you are working in and to never let others take away your credibility. You have worked hard to master your craft and need to ascertain what you are willing to negotiate at the time you begin your negotiations.

You are the author of your career so write the book that others really want to read and make it so valuable that they can't imagine their lives without it.

YOUR PURPOSE

Your passion is your purpose, and we are **blessed** to work in an industry that has a built-in purpose. We make another look and feel good. That in itself is a powerful purpose and one that you can choose to embrace.

If you are new to this industry you probably feel that powerful purpose inside you and fully embrace that you do help others to look and feel good. But if you have been in this industry for a while you may have lost that inner powerful sense of purpose.

Today we are going to look at finding your purpose in your beauty industry professional and give you a roadmap to embracing your purpose and sharing it with others. When you have a sense of purpose at work, you feel passionate, innovative, and committed. Your outward-looking focus is on serving others and giving all, you have to helping others look and feel good. If you are struggling to feel your purpose at work, then you will ultimately be destructive to your career and your career goals. If you don't know your purpose, then let's look at a few ways to help you focus on your mindset and find your passion and purpose.

Find Your Purpose

Life is short. You deserve a beauty industry career where you have a sense of purpose. But don't leave it up to others to help you find your passion and purpose. It is up to **you** to define and enact your purpose at work.

Top ways to find purpose:

- Know what motivates you
- Analyze your personal goals
- Find the niche that lets you be creative and have fun
- Discover ways you can help make your clients feel better
- Mentor, coach, and help others

Embrace Your Passion

Sometimes we don't even know that what we're doing each day is really our passion. If you started out in your beauty industry career to just make a living you might not know that you have a single area of expertise that inspires others. You might not recognize that you are already living your purpose but without passion. Passion is what others see in us and gives us a joyful experience at work. This is your lifelong career, and you must embrace the passion of your work to find the purpose in your life.

YOUR GOALS

Goal setting is a powerful process for achieving an ideal future for you and your beauty business, and it's essential for motivating yourself to turn the vision of your business future into reality.

The process of setting goals helps you choose where you want to go in life. By knowing precisely what you want to achieve, you know where you have to concentrate your efforts. It will also help you quickly spot the distractions that can, so easily, lead you astray in the wrong direction.

Many beauty industry professionals often feel as if they're adrift in their business goals. They work hard, but they don't seem to get anywhere or achieve the level of success that they dreamed about. **Dreams** are great to have but without goals and the process of setting goals, a dream is just a dream.

If you are feeling adrift, then you haven't spent enough time thinking about what you want from your business and you haven't laid out a path for your goals. After all, would you set out on a vacation with no real idea of your destination, how you're going to get there, and where you might be staying? Probably not!

It's time to learn how to set goals and how to achieve the outcomes that will fulfill your dreams.

Why?

Setting goals gives you long-term vision and short-term motivation. It helps you organize your time and enables you to see the achievements as they happen. It is the process of your business plan playing out right in front of you and you actually get to see the results.

You will need to set up clearly defined goals that you can measure and take pride in those goals as they unfold in your business. Having goals will help you gain self-confidence as you recognize your own abilities and the achievement of reaching your milestones.

How?

To begin start by creating categories in your business where you want to see results. Here is a small list of ideas. Ultimately you will need to decide what categories to put on your goals list and where they rank in importance.

- Career Improvements
- Continuing Education
- Relationship Building
- Social Media Engagement
- Salon Improvements
- Personal Improvements
- Financial Improvements
- Physical Improvements
- Customer Engagement
- Product Knowledge
- Product Sales
- Travel Goals
- Staff Building

Brainstorm your ideas, then select three ideas in each category that you want to achieve that best reflects what your goals are. Then set it aside and come back later and trim it down to be very focused on what really matters to you and the importance of each goal.

As you do this, make sure that the goals that you have set are ones that you genuinely want to achieve, consider what you want.

Once you've decided on your first set of goals, keep the process going by reviewing and updating your list as things change. Periodically review the longer-term goals in each category and modify them to reflect your changing priorities and experience. Add the review process to your monthly calendar and take time to review and adjust.

S.M.A.R.T. Goal Setting

A useful way of making goals more powerful is to use the S.M.A.R.T. Goals approach.

- S – Specific (or Significant).
- M – Measurable (or Meaningful).
- A – Attainable (or Action-Oriented).
- R – Relevant (or Rewarding).
- T – Time-bound (or Trackable).

For example, instead of having a goal to open a salon by 2027 use the SMART goal approach and write down small goals that would help you get to the end goal. To open a salon by 2027 I will need to do xxxxx steps to get there.

When you've achieved a goal, take the time to enjoy the satisfaction of having done so. Absorb the implications of the goal achievement and observe the progress that you've made towards other goals.

If the goal was a significant one, reward yourself appropriately and celebrate with those around you with whom you have shared your goals with. Saying your goals out loud to someone can help you become accountable to that person and you will be more likely to work hard toward that goal.

With the experience of having achieved this goal, review the rest of your goal plans:

- If you achieved the goal too easily, make your next goal harder.
- If the goal took a dispiriting length of time to achieve, make the next goal a little easier.
- If you learned something that would lead you to change other goals, do so.
- If you noticed a deficit in your skills despite achieving the goal, decide whether to set goals to fix this.

Example

For her New Year's Resolution, Lara has decided to think about what she really wants to do with her life.

Her lifetime goals are as follows:

- **Career** – "To be the lead stylist of the salon that I work for."
- **Artistic** – "To keep working on my styling skills and attend selective training and receive 4 certifications of expertise. Ultimately, I want to have my own hair show where I can showcase my work to others"
- **Physical** – "To run a marathon."

Now that Lara has listed her goals, she then breaks down each one into smaller, more manageable goals.

Let's take a closer look at how she might break down her lifetime career goal.

- **Five-year goal:** "Become a lead stylist and a managing partner."
- **One-year goal:** "Volunteer for projects that matter in my local community."
- **Six-month goal:** "Register for upcoming salon skill training and earn 4 certificates of completion."
- **One-month goal:** "Talk to the current manager to determine what skills are needed to do the job."
- **One-week goal:** "Book 5 extra hair color treatments."

As you can see from this example, breaking big goals down into smaller, more manageable goals makes it far easier to see how the goal will get accomplished.

Key Points

Goal setting is an important method for:

- Deciding what you want to achieve in your life.
- Separating what's important from what's irrelevant, or a distraction.
- Motivating yourself.
- Building your self-confidence, based on successful achievement of goals.

Set your lifetime goals first. Then, set a five-year plan of smaller goals that you need to complete if you are to reach your lifetime plan. Keep the process going by regularly reviewing and updating your goals. And remember to take time to enjoy the satisfaction of achieving your goals when you do so.

If you don't already set goals, do so, starting now. As you make this technique part of your life, you'll find your career accelerating, and you'll wonder how you did without it!

YOUR RELATIONSHIPS

Building relationships will prove to be your greatest asset as you venture out into your new business and the power of attraction marketing can skyrocket your business.

What does building relationships really mean and how can it get you bigger profits in your business?

In truth, the best part of your new career will be all the amazing relationships you get to make. The law of attraction says, "that you attract into your life whatever you think about." It is in these thoughts that we create our realities. Success can be a thought, but action is required to make this thought a truth. These thoughts and actions have to have specific positive outcomes to be considered a success. What you do with your thoughts will inherently lead you to take action in the direction you are trying to go, a successful beauty business!

Leave your Comfort Zone

To be successful in your new business you will need to add two skills.

Self-confidence and the ability to leave your **comfort zone**, the ability to step out into the world of building relationships and not just make acquaintances but building real connections with others by sharing your passion with them whilst appreciating their passions in life. The best way to do this is to help others solve their problems. Be a listening ear but also a problem-solving guru. You build true connections when you show others how to do things they struggle with or when you inspire them in some way.

True Connection

Reaching into the world of others makes true connections and to make these true connections will require personal contact. Here is the truth, to be a success and get to the top you will need to do that which 99% of the population is not willing to do!

Building relationships is a skill set and one that needs to be practiced daily just like you need to practice your professional beauty business techniques.

It may come easy for you to make friends; it may be second nature for you to reach out and touch someone's life and appreciate others. It may even be easy for you to pick up the phone and circumvent today's technology-based connections and make a personal connection. If this is true of you then I would say you are well on your way to success because these are the things you are going to have to do to be the best in your industry.

If it comes hard for you then you need to practice relationship building skills. I use a small personal group for my clients and customers. A place where I teach things and share tricks and tips. I also have a safe space for them to ask questions and share their tips and small secrets to help and inspire others.

Be brave and be fearless and I promise your relationships will blossom.

Be Fearless

To have a successful beauty business career takes courage and a fearless approach to life. You will need to learn how to appreciate others and learn to connect on a more personal level. This will require genuine glad-handing, truly getting to know people, and taking the time to learn about what others want and need. You are in the business of creating value for others and showing them the benefits of your business.

Never underestimate the power of you. You are and always will be the figurehead of your new business so be genuine and always be you. The power of self can carry its weight in gold and will give you the courage to continue on in your new business even when it's hard. It will be up to you to market yourself, build your clientele, and build the relationships that will continue to open up new opportunities.

The Do's of Building Strong & Powerful Relationships

Do: Ask for suggestions and favors!

It doesn't seem possible that asking for something will get you feedback and help build relationships, but the truth is we live in a positive society where people actually do want to help out other people. Once you ask for suggestions, feedback, or even favor the response will be quick and you will have begun to build a lasting relationship. I know it doesn't seem possible, but I once sent out a test on this. I asked 20 people I had done collaborations with if they could help me out. The response was almost instantaneous to my request and here is what I got in a return message: "How can I help." "Absolutely how can I be of assistance." It may not seem like it but we live in a world where others really do want to help out and everyone has a voice that they want to share. One of the best ways to ask for assistance is to get current and past clients to send you reviews. And here is how that conversation would go.

You: "Hey Jack I was wondering if I could ask a favor."

Jack: "Absolutely how can I help."

You: "I'm revamping my website and I need some customer reviews; would you be willing to write something short for me?"

Jack: "Sure, where can I send it?"

You: "Thank you, just email it here, and if you like add a photo of yourself."

Jack: "I will send it right over."

You "I really appreciate it, once again thank you."

This technique puts in in contact with past clients whom you may not have seen in quite a while and it gets you a review you can use on your social sites, your website, and anywhere else you may need it. People really do love to help and they are honored that you asked them for their assistance. We all want to share our voice, and this is a great way for you to connect and build stronger relationships.

Do: Support and share what others are doing!

I have many industry friends who are doing all types of creative endeavors. I openly support what they do, and I often share their posts and weblinks with my followers. I have a great friend who is an amazing female photographer who works with women to help them feel empowered. I often talk about her and her work in my live videos and I share her work on my social sites. In return, our relationship is very strong, and she recommends me often to her followers. I do this for people all the time and the benefit is it builds up a great deal of respect from others who know you recommend their services and from your followers who know you only recommend the best.

Do: Send random messages!

This **does not** mean send spam messages this means send connection messages. I often will send messages to people who I want to get to know better. It usually is because I saw something they posted or listed that they are interested in or when I know we have a common connection.

Here is how a connection message can appear. "Susan, I just saw your post about running, I have been running consistently for the past 5 years and I know it's hard to get started but once you do it can be such an amazing experience. I started because my husband is a marathon runner and I wanted to be able to enjoy his passion with him. My suggestion is to set a goal for yourself and then work towards that goal. If you ever need a running partner just let me know."

Find common ground and use it to build real and honest relationships.

Do: Share your story!

I have a private beauty group that I have had for years where my clients, my friends, and people who I personally know are located. I use this group to post tutorials and share valuable information that I think others might want to know. I also sometimes post-truths about myself that I wouldn't share anywhere else. Why? Well because I want my followers to know I am human. Sharing our story is how we find true connections with others and they get the opportunity to see our truths. Your story is valuable and may help others through their own struggles.

Do: Always be Professional!

I know this goes without saying but if you want to build a great clientele and make better sales then you need to always be a professional in your business. This means even in your personal life you are expected to behave with a manner of decorum that shows others your deep level of integrity. This also means you never talk business when you are out being social. There is a fine line between business conversation and personal conversation and knowing the difference is very important to building strong and lasting relationships.

5 Ways to Build Relationships that Last

1. Exceed Expectations: Your customers expect great products or services from you. You should continue to raise the bar on what your company offers. To put it simply, under promise, and over-deliver. When you impress customers, they keep coming back.

2. Ask for Feedback: Customer feedback helps you hone your customers' specific needs so you can find the best solutions to their problems. The better your offering meets their needs, the more your business will grow.

3. Connect: There are many online tools to help you connect with your customers. Ask questions and always respond to inquiries. Build customer relationships through your online presence. Do video tutorials, share tips and tricks and always follow-up.

4. Be Informative & Approachable: Regularly engage with your customers. Give them a link to your website or Facebook page where they can learn more about your product, services and tutorials.

5. Communicate: Rather than just telling customers about your business, have conversations with them. Find out what your customers need, then show them that you have a solution to their problem.

Network

Networking is one of the best ways to build your business quickly and it is the best way to start building relationships.

Attend Networking Events

Network at events where you can share your contact info, this is the most organic and easiest way to get your business out to people who may be looking for your special skills. And remember not everyone will need your services now but they more than likely will need your services in the future. *My Top Tip:* remember, it is not enough to just hand someone your business card, you need to get their contact info in return. If they don't have a business card ask if you can friend them on Facebook, then immediately send them your name and info as a message via Facebook, it is up to you to keep top of mind awareness of who you are and what services you have to offer. Try attending fashion events, makeup events, trade shows, chamber of commerce events, local business card social events, and always be a part of local and national bridal events. These events get you face to face with people who are looking for your services. You have a talent and a skill that others are looking for; you just have to be brave enough to talk about what you do and how you do it. Here is where I like to say, *"Be Fearless."*

Join Local Fundraisers

Support your local charity fundraising events by offering to sponsor a table or maybe by providing a gift certificate for their silent or live auction. Ask for a ticket to the event in return for your gift and then use this event to network in person. These events are usually filled with business professionals in your area and can have a very positive effect on your business.

Create Self Hosted Events

You might try hosting your own events. These can be a live in-person short intro class to specific styles or even a one-day course on certain techniques. These can be geared toward the everyday women looking to learn how to do natural cost-effective makeup routines or toward the bridal industry helping new brides learn how to do their own wedding day makeup. These could be directed at the younger generation of juniors who are starting to wear makeup and want to know some simple techniques. You decide whether these events are free or charge a minimal fee. Either way, you will be building lasting relationships while marketing your skills.

You could even have a 2-hour event on creating scented candles. All I know is that women like to gather, and women like to learn. Why do you think all these paint parties are so successful? Women are coming together and learning and enjoying themselves at the same time.

Create a Business Bookmark

I love this tip I found online in a makeup blog. Rather than simply creating an ordinary business card, create a business bookmark, and use it to insert into relevant books in the library, bookstore, or used bookstore. On this business bookmark, include your business information and a photo of you or one of your clients, try and make it personal. Then, head out and insert your business bookmarks into random pages of relevant books. For example, bridal books, wedding planning books, makeup books, wedding craft books, books about prom, modeling, photography, etc.

Join Free Online Sites

You know I don't recommend joining paid subscription sites like wedding wire or wedding pro (the cost is high and the ROI is low) but I do encourage you to join free space sites where you can create an online profile and list your skills and your location. These sites usually allow you to link your website or your Instagram account.

Model Mayhem is a site where creative professionals, such as photographers, models, makeup artists, hairstylists, and other beauty professionals can connect with one another. You can network with talented professionals in your area and work together to develop customers together. And, photographers, models, and interested clients can contact you for paid work through your profile. It's necessary to add value to the Model Mayhem community. Spend time creating a professionally written bio and uploading quality pictures. Also, take the initiative by reaching out to local talent to proactively network your way to success.

Thumbtack is an online beauty professional site where you the professional can list the services you provide, and clients seek a professional to accommodate their needs. This site will require you to fill out a bio and expect you to upload portfolio pictures, as well as your fees for services that you provide. Clients can come to you or you can go to your clients.

Online Networking

Website

Not all beauty professionals want to go out and build a website, but for some, it can be a great tool to get exposure in an overexposed industry. Building a website is not easy but there are lots of pre-made website hosting portals that have very good templates that you just fill in the photos and your info. This is also a great location for your portfolio to go. If you are tech-savvy, then a website should be on the top of your social media marketing list. I use WIX

Facebook

Setting up a Facebook page or group where you can attach photos of your work and a link to your website should be on the top of your list. Your Facebook page, not your personal profile page, is where you will invite your friends, family, and acquaintances from your personal Facebook page to like your business page and where you will start sharing your portfolio pictures and talking about the exciting world of your services. It is the place where you can share tips and tutorials and where you will put up your open for business sign. You are building your brand and Facebook is the perfect platform for you to begin building your business.

Instagram

This social site is important in building your image and your brand. Instagram is all about photos and #hashtags and using this platform is perfect for the budding beauty professional to build a following and a potential client base. One of the most important things to remember about Instagram, you need to use high-quality photos and build a brand that is easily recognized. Create consistent and recognizable images that when they appear your followers know it is one of yours.

Pinterest

This platform is a rising star on social media and is perfect for beauty professionals because its photo-based platform gives you the artist a place to showcase your talents. This site is great for your looks but can be used to post photo-based tips and tutorials. It is an easy way for you to share what you really admire and to follow others in the business who you admire. It also lets you link your website or portfolio to each photo, when a user clicks your picture they will be redirected back to your picture. Pinterest is a brilliant marketing tool right at your fingertips.

YouTube

YouTube is almost the perfect platform for up-and-coming beauty professionals. This video platform lets you take your business to a whole new level. TNW news says, "YouTube is huge. It has 1 billion users, it's the second-largest search engine, and over 300 hours of content are uploaded each minute. It is ubiquitous, generating 50 percent of its viewership via mobile, 80 percent of its traffic comes from outside the US, and the platform has been localized for 61 languages". So, with such a huge market, your business has the potential to reach a very large audience in a very short time. Creating demo videos, tutorial videos, and even just everyday life videos can really project your image to the masses. Think of YouTube as a way of getting your face and your brand out to the people you are connecting with. It's like talking to a room filled with people instead of just one person at a time.

Blogging

I love blogging and I currently have 4 websites where I blog and share beauty tips as well as life tips and other things I like to chat about. Start a blog and you can give tips and tricks on your area of expertise. You can talk about the issues that you are passionate about or the techniques that separate you from other beauty professionals. You can hone your writing skills by doing research about topics you want to discuss. Or you can become a guest blogger for other beauty sites and blogs. Utilize their avenue of people to build your network. It requires time to blog about your business and your interests, but I can guarantee that blogging helps you to find clarity in your business and gives you a platform to really get close to your fan base.

Traditional Marketing

Networking and Internet marketing will be the best tools you can use to start getting exposure for your business. But don't forget traditional marketing and the many other marketing tools you should have in your toolbox. These are the items you would use on hand and more in person or as inserts into gift baskets or mailers. Traditional marketing is still alive and well and should never be discounted. Here are a few traditional marketing tools that you should have in your marketing plan.

- Business Cards
- Blitz Cards
- Car Decals
- Brochures
- Banners
- Flyers

I could go on and on with marketing options for you to choose from but my advice to you would be this. In social media choose the platforms that you are comfortable with, then use them to showcase your passion for your craft and stay away from the selling aspect of marketing, just share your value-first content.

3 Step Social Media Approach

Lead with value, then make a call to action, and follow up with every person who engages with you.

- Post value-filled content
- Create a call to action
- Follow up every post engagement

In-Person Approach

In event marketing, you need to be present and outgoing and take the time to build relationships with people. Let them get to know you but take the time to get to know them. Follow up with every person you meet by connecting via social media and let them know how nice it was to meet them. Hand out your business cards but always get their contact info in return. Establish an immediate connection and it is up to you to follow up with them at a later date.

Traditional Marketing Approach

In traditional marketing, it is all about your brand. Getting your logo or brand out to the masses and becoming the leader in top-of-mind awareness when someone needs your services. Choose well the avenues of marketing in this arena but the paper is cheap, and your brand value is the wide exposure you get.

Follow up

No matter what you do to build your professional presence in the end it is always about the follow-up. The follow up declares your decision to stay connected to people and ultimately accomplish the goals you set out to achieve. It is you that will stand above the rest when you follow the rules of building your professional presence.

It takes more than a train case and a set of good brushes to be a successful makeup artist. It takes hard work, dedication to you, and your craft and patience to see it achieve its full potential.

YOUR BRAND

Creating your personal brand will take time and patience but it will be the recognition that defines you as a professional. Your top-of-mind awareness will determine your new career when the need arises for you as a beauty business professional. It will be up to you to create a brand that shows your true self and embodies your passion in a fun and professional way. While at the same time giving you an edge over your competition it will be up to you to keep your brand fresh and in the spotlight.

Why create a brand?

What will it accomplish and how does it help you get an edge up on your career?

Your personal brand will keep a connection between your profession and your person; it will be the factor that binds you and your skills with your audience. Think of all the professional beauty influencers whom you follow or admire? I bet with just their first name you know exactly what their brand is. Maybe even a logo or symbol will conjure up images of their face or one of their images. This is called a personal brand, sight recognition that brings you back to the name and face of a person and the services they provide.

How do you begin to create your personal brand? First, you take a very close look at how others see you right now and then determine how you want others to see you. My husband would call this an OV1 meaning where are you now and what is the road map of where you want to be.

- What reminds people of you?
- What are friends and family tagging you in on social media?
- What are others saying about you and your work?
- What are you passionate about that you can bring to your work?
- What are 5 things you think of when you think of yourself?
- What are 3 things you value and what to incorporate into your business?
- You may own a business, but you are the brand.

To determine your **personal brand,** you need to start a list and get others involved. Write down how you perceive yourself and your style of business or your business values. Then ask others how they perceive you. Then start to get more specific; what can you incorporate into your world and professional self that will create your brand.

Logo

Your logo will be a huge part of your brand. When deciding what to use make sure it is a reflection of you and how you want to be seen. Make it original and easy to read. Give it colors that stand out and use a font that is bold yet creative. Be original and be you.

Business Cards

Your business card should have your logo as well as your name, phone number, website, online portfolio, or social media site. Make it easy to read with fonts that are true to you and your brand. You should also have an electronic business card that can be sent through text, social media, or email. I attend a lot of parties and never carry my business card. I always ask others for their business card and when they ask for mine in return I say, "oh I have an electronic one can I just text it to you?" Bam! I've done two things. They now have my electronic business card and I have their contact information. I create my electronic business card in Canva and then keep it in a file on my phone. That way I don't even have to pay for printing costs!

Here is an example of my e-biz card

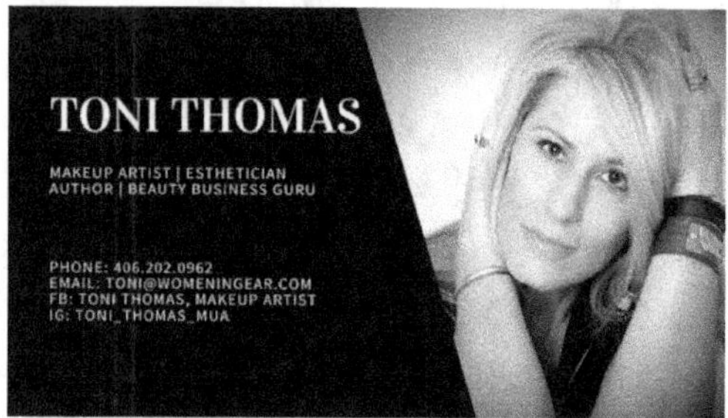

Videos

Building your brand through videos can be one of the fastest ways to get your personal brand out to the world. Be creative and fun but more importantly it is in your best interest to be consistent. It will be up to you to be unique, funny, original, and amazing. One fact to think about with videos, 78% of all videos are opened and if done well they are watched through to the end. The first rule of the video is you only have 8.25 seconds to grab the attention of your audience. It will be up to you to start your video with a great intro.

Building your brand is more than a look or a logo, it is an all-encompassing reflection of you and should be consistent on all of your marketing sites. A personal brand will encompass the complete package that is you the beauty professional. It will be up to you to create strong relationships, build credibility, and trust. One of the most important aspects of your brand will be to create professional relationships with your clients who know you are ethical and reliable. You will need to be connected to your brand as a constant in your everyday life. Consistency-Consistency-Consistency!

You are the author of your career so write the book that others really want to read and make it so valuable that they can't imagine their lives without it.

Marketing

Brand loyalty is an invaluable reward that you earn by truly caring for your followers. If you want your social media marketing to be effective, you need to be actively engaged with your loyal followers.

Social media follower counts are a distraction to you and your goals, so you need to focus on the brand, not the follower count or the like numbers. You are an important piece of the marketing strategy and it is your job to solve problems, give value, and get local level followers who are looking for your products and services.

I always get this feeling that having 10,000 followers on social media means you aren't really focusing on the important people who need what you have to offer. This type of huge social media exposure keeps you out of the loop of the local level exposure you want and need.

Brand loyalty is what really matters. This will naturally ensure long-term engagement on social media with the followers who are looking for what you have to offer.

Fortunately, there are several strategies that can help you build customer loyalty and to enhance your brand's online image.

Here are six ways to increase your brand loyalty on social media.

In today's highly competitive market, brand loyalty is incredibly hard to come by.

Resistance to the competition. Follower numbers may increase new followers' perception of your brand, but it's the loyal followers who add real value in the long run of your beauty business. And unless you sell products globally you want local brand loyalty and engagement.

Enthusiasm and engagement. A thousand loyal followers are worth far more than 10,000 indifferent followers. Loyal followers are more likely to interact with your posts and create meaningful conversations. Real engagement is more valuable to your online image and SEO than follower count.

Advocacy – Loyal social media followers are high potential brand advocates. They're very likely to talk about your brand positively, even without persuasion. The right social media campaign can turn several loyal fans into invaluable messengers spreading awareness about your brand.

Create a smart social media strategy: You can't rely only on your advertising, marketing, and sales strategies to carry you through social media because each platform comes with its unique opportunities and intricacies.

Social media marketing has moved beyond the simple acts of posting and interaction to include advertising, marketing, lead generation, selling, and support combined.

It's essential to create a strategy that includes a cohesive plan for PR, SEO, and prospect mining to keep up with your competition.

When focusing on your brand loyalty, ask what value you can create for your fans on social media. The answer you come up with needs to be powerful enough to inspire your fans to be loyal. It's a good idea to research your competition when creating your social media strategy.

Create quality content: To inspire brand loyalty on social media, you need to share valuable content or useful content with your followers.

The way you present your content and the formats you choose also matter. In terms of metrics, shares, likes, comments, and click-throughs.

Visual content gets noticed and shared more via social networks, so it's important to factor them in when planning your social media content. Use infographics, videos, screenshots, graphs, and visual aids where possible, to make your content more striking and memorable. For beauty business professionals before and after photos are a great way to get your work and your brand out to your followers. Also, ensure that your content is branded, with your logo, colors, and chosen font consistently used on everything you share.

Share your truth: Followers want to interact with real people, not robots or automated content. Ensure that you don't sideline personal interactions as something to do when you have time.

Prioritize personal interactions and use them to show fans your personality. The warmth will keep your followers coming back for more interactions with you.

Some brands use common values and interests to connect with people. For instance, if you enjoy hiking, you can make the occasional hiking-reference on your social posts, or talk about current events related to it.

Cause based social campaigns are another way to connect with your audience and their values. Share what you are passionate about and where you volunteer your time.

Consistency: People associate others with their strongest personality traits. That's what you remember about people and that's what lingers on your mind. As a brand, it's important to create and consistently display favorable personality traits to build familiarity among people.

These traits can be expressed through content sharing and conversations you have with people. If your routine includes blog content promotion, answering questions related to your industry, and commenting on other people's shares, each of those tasks should be completed in the same voice.

Answer and acknowledge: People want to be acknowledged. If you consistently respond to their queries with useful, detailed answers, you can earn their respect. This is probably what you will notice if you look at the historic footprint left by any social media influencer.

You don't have to limit answers to your fans. You can expand your exposure by finding questions asked by anyone and answering them. Use keywords related to your specific beauty industry and your location as search queries to find questions and respond to them with precise and concise answers. Remember to acknowledge any responses you receive and see the conversations through.

Be human: Your followers are most certainly creating content of their own and participating in conversations, possibly related to your industry. You can use social media monitoring to find them and share their content if they are share-worthy. By doing this, you not only earn the loyalty of those followers but encourage other followers to share content related to your brand.

Another great way of managing relationships with followers is through Twitter lists. Add followers who have similar levels of engagement with your brand in Twitter lists and visit your lists once a week to interact with them. Finally, don't forget the rewards. The right rewards for the best of your followers can be powerful in earning their loyalty. Many brands have loyalty programs to extend to the best of their fans.

You need to be human to connect with your fans.

Simply pushing content doesn't suffice. You have to move beyond that effort to make a lasting impression on your customers and social media followers.

Dress for Success and Exude Confidence

One of my **biggest** pet peeves is working with other beauty industry professionals who show up late for a gig or even worse show up to a gig looking like they just rolled out of bed. Being comfortable in this industry is important but looking sloppy to be comfortable is just unacceptable. I am not pointing any fingers but part of working in the beauty industry and building your brand is looking your best and making sure you are dressed for success.

Dressing for success to me means looking good and feeling confident. Clothes have the ability to make us feel confident in any situation and when you dress well you feel good.

When we dress nice, we feel good and we get an extra boost of confidence this in turn helps us to have better posture, and when we feel good we tend to look people in the eye and exude confidence.

Dressing well doesn't have to cost a fortune. Implementing a few key pieces into your wardrobe can give you the added confidence boost you need and will help you look fabulous and well put together.

I know in this industry we all want to be comfortable, let's be honest we are on our feet all day, working hard moving around a lot, and we want to wear clothes that feel good. But trying to dress comfortably doesn't mean we need to sacrifice looking fabulous. There are loads of options for you as a working beauty industry professional.

Brand Your Look

In an industry filled with so many artists and beautiful people, I think the best way to start your career is to have a branded look. A branded look means you incorporate signature pieces into your wardrobe that people automatically recognize as you.

Do you love a certain hat? Do you like to wear knee boots to work? Do you have a favorite piece of jewelry or style of jewelry that you often wear? Do you like to wear wrap sweaters or skirts? I am of the belief that wearing black every day is not a brand it's just the same look everyone else in your industry is wearing. Be bold! Be Brave! Be Unique and find a signature piece to add to your wardrobe that becomes a part of your brand.

If you choose to wear jeans to work, then dress them up with boots or a beautiful scarf. Jeans can be very gorgeous if you add a signature sweater, hat, or a beautiful chunky piece of jewelry.

I recommend black of course for beauty professionals but add a signature color piece to your look. Wear a great belt that compliments your look and is bold enough to stand out on its own. Throw a great blazer over a signature quote t-shirt as your added accessory. I love all the new hat styles available today. Hats can really give you a signature look. If you aren't into hats, then be creative and make your jewelry your stand-out signature look.

Whatever you choose to do with your work style be specific in your decisions and have purpose in your style.

Brand loyalty is an invaluable reward that you earn by truly caring for your followers.

YOUR MARKETING

Your marketing strategy should be long-term, forward-looking, and consistent with your brand. It should be implemented with the purpose of your beauty business. The fundamental goal of marketing is to find clients and achieve a sustainable client base by using different marketing tools available to you. Strategic marketing involves an analysis of your business plan and a good understanding of your target audience.

Identify Your Target Audience

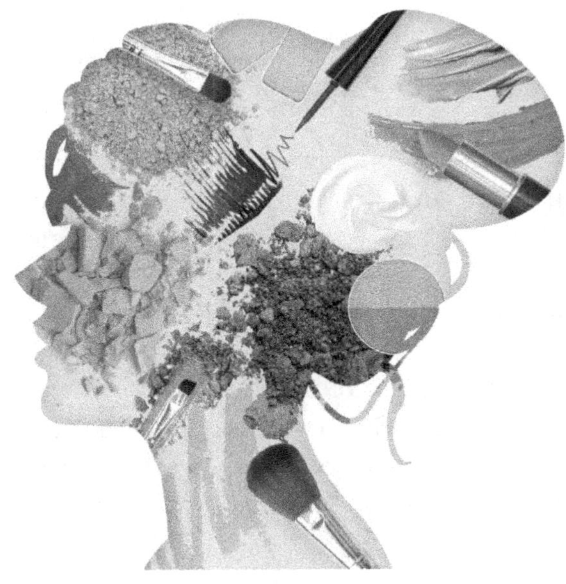

Your target market is the type of person you think will buy your service or the kind of person to whom your products and services are useful. A person who in fact is already looking your you but they just haven't found you yet.

Knowing your target market is essential to your beauty business, as it helps you to tailor your advertising and marketing to that audience, thus maximizing the number of likely clients who become aware of your services. After all, it's no-good spending hard-earned advertising revenue on trying to woo consumers who do not need your product and have little intention of buying it!

Who is your target client and what do they look like? Where do they currently go now for their services and how much are they spending?

Who is your perfect client and what do they look like?

What are their wants and needs and what problems do they have that you can solve?

How do you create a target customer profile to help you in your marketing approach?

A Customer Persona

You need to develop a perfect client persona. This is achieved by creating an 'ideal' customer who represents a particular type of individual you want to serve and help to solve their problems.

You may develop a client persona based on your business approach. Maybe you are an organic product user who is very eco-conscience. Or you might build a persona for younger customers who primarily engage with your business via social media and YouTube tutorials. Maybe you have a smart salon where everything is geared toward customer awareness.

When creating a persona, think about the demographics but also go a little deeper. What motivates your audience? What do they want, and what problems do they need solving?

You may end up with a single persona or a few. Remember, each persona represents a group of individuals, not one client but many. Once you've completed your personas, write down the details and include them in your branding, and use them in your marketing strategies.

Align Your Values

Once you've established your personas, it's all about aligning your business with their values and interests. This means being the voice that your target customers want, need, and enjoy hearing.

You must be authentic. The trick is to find a way of meeting the needs of your audience with your own values and beliefs. You need to align your values with those of your prospective clients.

You should also make an effort to incorporate affinity topics into your marketing content. Affinity topics are subjects that don't obviously fall within the purview of traditional beauty content, but that share a strong link with your industry or have some kind of crossover.

For instance, beauty often goes hand in hand with fashion, so you should think about creating content around this. Likewise, beauty is heavily associated with art, and there's a big chance that fans of art will be interested in your beauty business.

Publish the Right Content

Different platforms are suited to different types of content and will be viewed by different users. For instance, long-form content is better suited to blogs, while before/after beauty photos fit much more comfortably on your beauty business Instagram page and stories. Tailoring your content to a platform is the key to success.

There are also significant differences between social platforms. Different demographics prefer certain networks, and you'll need to work out your target audience's favorite channels if you want your social media marketing to be effective.

Engage

Now that you understand the needs of your target audience, you have to show how your services can meet their needs. List the features and benefits of your services, and don't be shy about making a song and dance over specialist ingredients, customer reviews, or your own industry knowledge.

Your ongoing success is dependent on your ability to promote new services or products and to tap into emerging trends. The beauty industry is built on constant reinvention and innovation; customers are always looking for the 'next big thing,' and you need to meet this demand.

Know Your Audience

It's important to know that customers, your target audience and never take them for granted. They're always growing, developing, and evolving. You need to follow suit and do the same.

If you're to keep up with the needs of your customers, you must keep an eye on the available data, and review your strategy when you need to. Don't lose out because you're sticking with outdated ideas about who your target audience is and what do they want? How can you maximize the efficiency of your marketing strategy by keeping it fresh?

A target audience allows you to fine-tune your marketing strategy and get the biggest bang for your buck when it comes to your promotions.

Social Media is challenging on so many levels, with constant change new algorithms, and updates that take you back to square one. But with a few key strategies, you can grow your brand and your profits using your social media accounts.

Instagram

The best way to approach your Instagram account is to treat it like a mini website!

Would you put personal photos of you at the beach on your website? Would you put a less than stellar photo up on your website? Would you use inappropriate language or show inappropriate images on your website?

No, you wouldn't! So, let's start with how your Instagram **should look**.

CREATE AN AMAZING PROFILE BIO

Your Instagram bio is your business card, portfolio, and mini website all in one. You have just seconds to make a great first impression, so you need to focus on your Instagram bio and make sure it's fully equipped to convert Instagram visitors into followers.

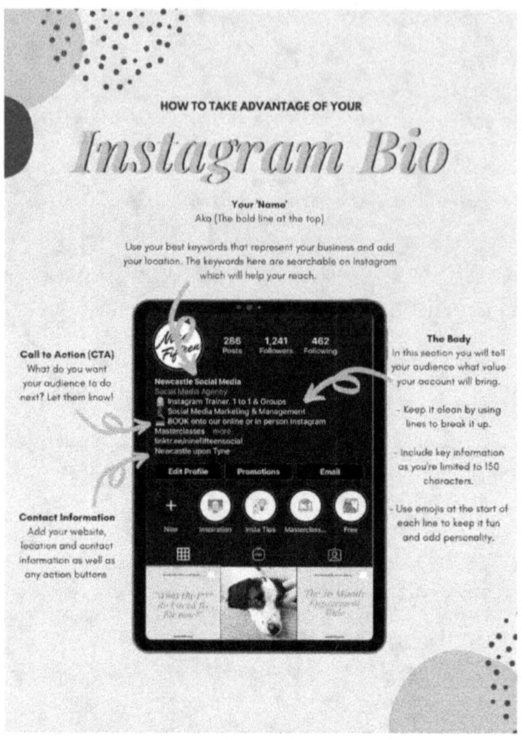

TREAT YOUR INSTAGRAM LIKE YOUR OWN MINI-WEBSITE

This is a business page, not a personal page. If you want to change your personal page to a biz page go to your settings and click "Switch to Professional Account". This way, you can get access to insights about your account performance, follower habits, and publicly share contact options on your profile bio so potential clients know where they can reach you.

Insights on Instagram allow you to filter your posts in order to see what received the most engagement, reach, impressions, shares, follows, and more. It even provides information about your followers and what times/days they are most active on your profile.

This way, you can begin to analyze what types of posts perform the best and get a better understanding of what your audience is responding to, as well as what kind of content *isn't* moving the needle. For example, if all of your drastic client haircut pictures all receive more engagement and reach than updos, you can assume that your audience really loves transformation content.

PROVIDE QUALITY CONTENT AND BE CONSISTENT

Imagine a profile that shares content 5x a week, but their photos are not all that great. Some are blurry, you can see their messy work area in the background, they overuse filters, their captions have grammar errors, and there's no consistency. This is a bad way to approach your Instagram account.

Now imagine a profile that shares content only 3x a week, but their posts are **amazing**. In fact, you can't help but like and comment on all of their pictures, you love the diversity in their posts, the photos are all on consistent backgrounds, and you're so inspired by their page that they're on your list of people that make you think, "I wish my professional profile was like theirs."

Well, take a play from their playbook! Emulate what you see by your favorite Instagrammer!

It's better to post less frequently and have an inspiring, mesmerizing profile that wins you, new clients, than to post as often as possible with completely sub-par content. So, what's it really mean to have quality content?

There are a few sure-fire ways to make your content stand out for your work, skills, personality, and professionalism.

A CLEAN BACKGROUND

Taking pictures at your station, your salon, your treatment room? Make sure you've cleaned it up: no products splayed about and move your client's water glass out of the way. You want to make it look as presentable as possible as if a new client were to be starting their service. If there's something lingering in the background, chances are your audience will fixate on that rather than your masterpiece.

Rather than taking pictures at your station, designating a plain wall in your location where you can take photos. A plain wall will have nothing that distracts the viewer, allowing them to focus all of their attention on the new look you're presenting or the before and after you want to show.

DON'T JUST TAKE ONE PICTURE

Not two. Not five. Take a bunch. This way, once you're ready to share on your professional Instagram, you will end up with enough photos to choose from. You only have a few minutes between your client leaving and your next appointment starting. Make taking a number of pictures part of your regular routine with every client. Try taking pictures in different ways, like:

From different distances away, try some shots closer up, some further back, and you'll begin to see what looks best for what kinds of looks.

- Different views of the hair, such as the client from the front, back, and side. Did you cut some new, beautiful layers or add some peekaboo colors? You want your audience to see that!
- Encourage your client to do different things, like run their hands through their hair, or hold up their newly chopped off 10-inch ponytail.
- Did you do a wispy lash extension? Take a before and after.
- Did you create an amazing bridal makeup look? Take a before and after but be sure to post after the wedding not before!
- Did you create an amazing new updo? Share it.

You'll quickly begin to get in touch with your own personal style, figuring out what aesthetically looks best on your page and what people respond to most. Do you get more engagement on close up photos? Action shots?

Plus, now you have a variety to pick from, rather than only having two choices and you can't use either because they both have a reflection from your ring light. *Not* quality content.

MAKE SURE YOUR CLIENTS SMILE!

Have fun with your clients. They are after all your best advertisement and your best referral source. You want to show all of your viewers how jazzed your clients are about their new looks, and how they'll be just as thrilled when they come to see you next.

While we typically focus on smiles, currently during COVID regulations, try having clients leave their masks on. You may not think it looks pretty, but it shows your dedication to the health and safety of your clients. **Big win.**

BEFORE AND AFTER PICTURES

This is the best way to show clients the magic that you create. A beautiful "after" shot is one thing, but when you can pair it with how drastic the change was compared to their "before" look, your audience will really be able to see your talent. Either post them side by side together as one photo or feature them in a carousel image with the new hair first and the old hair second.

Remember, though: if you post them as one photo, make sure that aside from the hair, the pictures look identical. The photos are taken from the same distance, at the same place, etc. Most importantly, take off any robe or cape they have on from the appointment (this goes for *all* client photos you take)!

CAROUSEL IMAGES

Did you know carousel posts perform better than a standard single photo? This is because they allow you to share more detailed and related content with your audience. Think of different ways you can share the same look in more than one photo—you could show pictures throughout the service. You could even use carousel images as a way to share what products and tools you used, especially if it's a newly launched product or something involved in a marketing promotion. Or even if it's just your fave go-to! Once a client sees the volume you created with the texturizing spray you shared, they'll immediately be asking for it the next time they see you. Ca-Ching, commission!

TUTORIALS/HOW-TO VIDEOS

Like carousels, video posts perform much better than one still image. And there's no better way to demonstrate your skills than through tutorials and how-to videos on your professional Instagram.

We all know that tutorials are *huge* in beauty (how do you think we finally got our winged liner down?), offering you an instant opportunity to attract more viewers, followers, and customers. By teaching people how to achieve different styles or how to use different products, you're proving you're a real expert. You know everything there is to know about hair, and you're going to show and teach them.

Videos are also a great way to demonstrate and show the genuine, authentic you! Through pictures of clients, people get to know your stellar work as a hairdresser, but they don't know you as a person. By sharing videos that feature you, they'll feel even more connected and likely to book an appointment with you—they know the *real you* now! They know you're fun, knowledgeable, personable, and that spending an hour or two with you will be the highlight of their day.

CLIENT SELFIES

Encourage your selfie-taking clients to either post their photos or text them to you so you have access to use them as well. Client selfies can be used either as a post or in a story, though we do recommend if they post it as a story and include GIFs/stickers/writing, etc., that you use it as a story as well. Don't throw off your clean, professional profile by sharing a picture that's been doodled on.

Think of client selfies as the Instagram version of a positive review. People listen to other people and trust the recommendations given to them by those they know. If they're willing to share their new hair with their followers and tag you in it, you know that means they're thrilled with their new look and love having you as their hairdresser.

Make sure they tag you; then you can repost the photo to your own story, and whoever sees your client's story will have access to your profile and see even more examples of your work. Bam. You just got some new clients.

STORIES

Stories are a great place to share your behind-the-scenes photos, videos, or Boomerangs that you may not want to feature on your main feed, but give followers exclusive insight into your day at the salon. Much like video tutorials, stories help to provide a better idea of who *you* are and let potential clients get to know you on a more personal level. You could share:

- You and your teammates during training to show viewers you're always advancing your skills.
- Retail information, like what your favorite products are, what new products are available, or any marketing promotions.
- Reposts of client stories with your own added sentiments. Don't just repost their story and leave it—add a thank you, a note about how great they look, etc.

- Repost stories from businesses surrounding your salon. When you support other businesses, they often return the favor.
- Post a photo, video, or Boomerang of you being silly with some of your favorite clients.
- Use polls and questionnaires. For example, use a poll to find out what kind of how-to video people want to see next, or have them ask product questions using the questionnaire feature.
- Announce last-minute appointment opportunities if you've had a cancellation.

When posting stories, be sure to provide as much information as possible: tag the people in it, tag the retail featured, tag your location, and of course, tag your salon!

To learn more, check out the Ninefifteen Instagram Masterclass. An **email marketing campaign** can add a great deal to your social media marketing campaigns.

Email is a totally different approach and can get you a little closer and more personal with your clients, followers, and fans.

I personally love email marketing because I can add more content and get more personal with those who I know what the services, products, and valuable information that I have to share.

What is Email Marketing?

An **email marketing campaign** is an email sent from a business to customers or prospects. A successful email marketing campaign will get the recipients to take action, engage with your business, and help you to **get more leads and sales**.

One of the advantages of email marketing is that people still use email widely.

This makes email marketing the perfect tool for building client relationships to help with leads and sales.

But before you begin there are a few steps you need to implement.

Build an Email List

The most successful email marketing campaigns start with an email list. The best way to build a targeted email list is to **convert your website visitors into subscribers**.

But did you know that on average, 80% of your website visitors will leave your site for good, without signing up for your newsletter?

That's why we recommend using exit-intent popups to convert those abandoning visitors into subscribers and customers.

Set Realistic Goals

All good marketing starts with setting goals, and email marketing is no different. To run a successful email marketing campaign, think about what you want to achieve. Typical goals for an email marketing campaign include:

- **Welcoming new subscribers** and telling them about your business and values so you start to build a relationship with them.
- **Boosting engagement** with your content and your business, whether that's promoting a webinar or trying to make an initial sale.
- **Nurturing existing subscribers** by providing something they'll value.
- **Re-engaging subscribers** who haven't been particularly active.
- **Segmenting your subscribers** so you can send more targeted email marketing campaigns.

Email Campaign Types

It's important to understand the different types of email campaigns that you can send.

Promotional emails: Talk about offers and sales and are self-promotional and don't get much reaction.

Relationship emails: Give your subscribers that value content you've promised, like weekly tips & tricks, a free gift, relevant information they can actually use.

Transaction emails: Triggered by subscribers' actions and relate to an action they've taken on your site.

Know Your Customers & Plan Your Emails

If you've been doing email marketing for a while, you'll likely know who your audience is. If you're just getting started, you'll have to make some educated guesses so you can target your content. Don't worry; you'll start collecting subscriber info the minute you send your first campaign, so next time around, you'll have real data to work with.

Once you know your goals, email type, and audience and you've attracted people onto your list with targeted options, it's time to plan your email marketing campaign.

A good approach is to know:

- Email frequency
- Ideas for content
- The main action you want subscribers to take (such as signing up for an event, following you on social media, buying a product)

Kuno Creative says that in creating your emails you need to make them timely, relevant, interesting, and valuable.

For example, many companies' welcome new subscribers with a short email series to help them get to know their products and services.

Try a series of 4 emails.

The email subject lines are:

1.   Welcome to (Your Business)
2.   What do you need to get done this week?
3.   Plan your day with (Your Business)
4.   Hit your next deadline

The first is a welcome email. Three days later, there's another email asking what you need to get done and encouraging you to start using the product. Two days later, there's an email talking about the Asana dashboard. The series ends with an email two days later, which highlights the calendar view.

Don't overwhelm your subscribers by emailing too often. That will send them straight to the spam button. Instead, stick to the schedule you've told them about, so they know what to expect.

Don't be afraid to ask for subscriber input on email scheduling via a poll or survey. You can also offer an "opt down" option for those who love your emails but don't want to get them as often.

Once you've outlined your email plan, it's time to start writing.

Email Content

Content to consider for your email:

- **A personal story**. Being human never hurts a company and often helps people make an emotional connection. Some of the most successful emails we've seen use this technique.

- **Something of value to your readers**. That can be a piece of content, some useful information, or the resource you're promoting. Make it clear how this will help them.
- **A poll, survey, GIF, or video**, all of which are proven to keep readers more engaged.

I can't tell you how important it is for you to follow up on every email you get back from a client, customer, fan, or potential client.

Traditional Marketing Tools

I love traditional marketing it has worked for hundreds of years and if done right can still work today. As a beauty business professional traditional marketing is great for local business owners who want to target their local audience. Did you know a radio ad can be more effective than months of social media marketing? One well-placed press release can get your phone ringing off the hook.

Press Release

I am a huge fan of press releases. I use them when I open a new business or if I am doing something that I know is newsworthy. If you have never done a press release you may not know their value, but the best part of a press release is that it is free and can get you big returns. Here is a great article from Just Reach Out on how to write and submit a press release.

Direct Mail Marketing

Direct mail is making a real comeback. Once upon a time, people would tag it as a snail mail and shrink away. But now, direct mail scores on creativity, personalizing and targeting a particular audience. Direct mail is not just easier to understand, it also has a greater power to influence readers. Brand recall is way higher in research studies where direct mail as compared to other marketing methods like email. Faster response rates, more purchases and greater ease of retrieval make good old-fashioned direct mail the real deal in new-age marketing. The #1 direct mail marketing can be a simple as sending a thank you postcard to your customers once a year or have an open house where you invite only your customers who utilize your services. Or give a direct mail discount to customers who refer a friend.

Consider why the pen may be mightier than the sword when it comes to marketing. Direct mail in the beauty industry can evoke a higher response rate. Why? Because not many beauty professionals are utilizing direct mail to market their business. Here is a great article from Lucid Press on how to utilize direct mail marketing.

Flyers and Brochures

Brick and mortar establishments, on-location, or studios are just some of the places where flyers and brochures can come in handy. These are still the most widely preferred methods for special discounts and offers. Consider the value of business cards that directly introduce a business to the client. Traditional marketing that is face-to-face is way more connective and interactive.

Don't underestimate the power of hand-outs to bring your business new growth opportunities. Direct mail and business cards also elicit emotional reactions and are more easily absorbed than words on a screen. Message mediums like these evoke strong responses and greater reach for marketers.

Print Ads

Print marketing is not dying; it is merely evolving. Social media penetration has only made print media more distinctive. Newspapers and magazines are visible on digital mediums and the smartphone could well be a bonus for print ads.

Event Marketing

During the olden days, traditional copyright marketing ruled the roost; nowadays, the game is all about generating a buzz. While the power of a persuasive copy should be ignored at your own peril, traditional marketing now incorporates event marketing with a difference. Networking is the key to attracting top talent besides marketing products and services. Online marketing cannot bridge this divide.

I personally do not utilize any paid platforms ie: weddingwire or weddingpro for my business the return on investment is way too low. I prefer to utilize local events that get me face to face contact with potential clients. One of my businesses is my team of on-location bridal makeup artists. We travel to the event location and do bridal party make up. So, my team and I attend as many bridal fairs as possible in our chosen locations and get the opportunity to showcase our portfolio as well as do demonstrations. At the event, I gave a small pre-booking discount if a bride makes a small deposit and books with us at the event. This usually guarantees my team of makeup artists is usually booked out for 12 months. The return on the cost of the event is small compared to the bookings we get at the event. Plus, as an added bonus I receive the email list of all the attendees. Win-Win!

The core value a sale generates is the service. Just as no amount of good marketing can sell a bad product, the reverse holds true as well. Marketing is an art that derives its value from traditional techniques because this is the way it has always been done.

From baby boomers to Gen-X, and Gen-Y, Millennial to Swinging Sixties, traditional marketing covers a lot of ground. While digital marketing is continuing to gain ground, traditional marketing techniques remain an important secret weapon for interactive, face-to-face, and skilled marketing.

Maximize Your potential.

1. Create business cards with a $5 off coupon on the back of the card. Place these business cards at your local women's gym. Women who go to gyms are great potential clients because they are already trying to look their best.
2. Partner up with wedding planners or wedding photographers and ask them to recommend you to upcoming brides. Brides often get eyelash extensions put on for their wedding and maybe they will become repeat customers.
3. Create a good atmosphere. Provide a quiet, peaceful, clean environment for your client to relax in while they are getting their lashes done. Getting lashes put on should be an experience the client enjoys.
4. Give away a full set of new eyelash extensions to a charity auction. You will possibly create a repeat customer who will come back for fills and they will talk about their new lashes with their friends and family.
5. Do 2 to 5 full sets of eyelash extensions for free. Pick people who work or play around other potential clients. They will become free advertising for you.
6. Offer a "Mother & Daughter Discount" to any mother and daughter that makes an eyelash extension appointment within the same day or week.
7. Advertise at local colleges and give a "Student Discount" for full sets.
8. Educate your clients on proper lash care. If your client takes care of their lashes then they will love them. If your client loves their lashes then they will talk about them and they will give your name to other potential clients.
9. If you see a slow week coming up advertise a 2 or 3-day sale where you lower your full set price. This will give you a boost in new clients to fill the openings during the slow week.

10. Start a loyalty card program. Have loyalty cards printed up that indicate after a certain number of visits a client can get a flat amount off an eyelash extension fill?

11. Give a client your business card with her name on it and initial it. Tell the client that if a new client comes in with that business card you will give her a discount on her next fill.

12. Offer gift certificates and advertise them to your existing clients as a great gift for birthdays and holidays.

13. If you have a smartphone, get a card reader for your phone and offer this payment option to your clients. The more payment options you have the more willing a customer is to give you their business.

14. Have too many clients? Raise your prices. You will lose a few clients at first, but you will keep many because they like your work and you will gain many new clients that will pay your new prices.

15. Sponsor an event at the local college and provide a flyer explaining what eyelash extensions are. Young women are interested in eyelash extensions, they just don't know where to get them or what exactly eyelash extensions are.

The bottom line is this is your beauty business and no one but you can make it a success. With hard work, commitment, executable techniques and consistent follow through you can be a superstar in your industry.

ABOUT THE AUTHOR

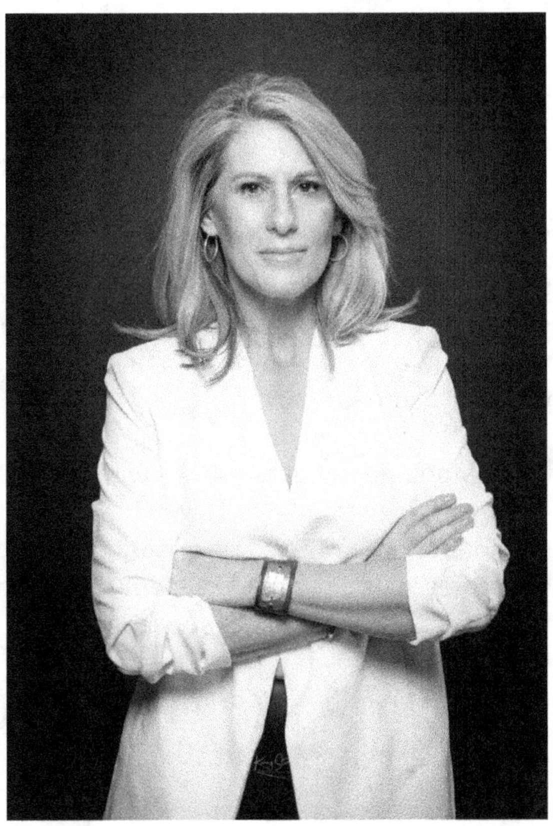

Toni Thomas is an award-winning beauty industry professional, international makeup artist, author of several beauty industry books, founder of The Beauty Academy, and the creative director of Sol Style Magazine.

Her makeup artistry has been featured in several fashion publications, on the runway of New York Fashion Week, and on national television for Fox News Network and ABC News.

As a beauty industry leader, she has spent her entire career in and around the beauty business working with some of today's most influential creators. Her focus is on projects that inspire creativity and make a difference to the world around her. She has committed her life to the beauty industry and lives each day working on her creative passions.

As a leader in the beauty industry guiding other beauty industry professionals in building their beauty businesses, she truly enjoys working with those who share her vision. She enjoys teaching beauty business skills to those who are willing to take a leap of faith in their creative careers. As one of the pioneers for quality online beauty education, she is committed to all aspects of an industry that has lacked credibility for far too long.

Born and raised in Montana, she now travels with her husband between their home in the mountains of Montana and their home in Virginia. Her passion to make others feel beautiful and inspiring beauty business professionals has made a global impact on the world of business, makeup artistry, and the beauty industry.

You can find more about her 'Rock Your Beauty Biz' course online Toni-Thomas.org

www.ingramcontent.com/pod-product-compliance
Lightning Source LLC
Chambersburg PA
CBHW070817240726
48654CB00007B/388